PUBLIC HEALTH AND ECONOMIC RESILIENCE: IMPLICATIONS FOR BUSINESS, GOVERNMENT, AND SOCIETY

DR BHARATH J

Made with ♥ on the Notion Press Platform
www.notionpress.com

This book is dedicated to all the public health professionals, economic experts, and policymakers who have tirelessly worked towards creating a healthier and more resilient society. Your unwavering commitment to the well-being of individuals and communities, especially during times of crisis, is truly admirable.

We also dedicate this book to all the business leaders who have recognized the importance of public health and economic resilience in achieving sustainable growth and development. Your proactive efforts towards building a healthier and more resilient business environment are inspiring.

Finally, we dedicate this book to all the individuals and communities who have been affected by public health and economic challenges. Your resilience and perseverance in the face of adversity serve as a reminder of the importance of collaboration and collective action towards a healthier and more equitable future.

May this book inspire and inform all those who are working towards building a healthier and more resilient society.

Contents

Foreword

Public Health and Economic Resilience are two crucial pillars of a thriving society. The COVID-19 pandemic has brought to light the significant interplay between these two fields and highlighted the need for a better understanding of their implications for businesses, governments, and society as a whole.

This book, titled "Public Health and Economic Resilience: Implications for Business, Government, and Society," presents a comprehensive analysis of the complex relationship between public health and economic resilience. The authors have done an excellent job of exploring the impact of public health policies and economic systems on each other, highlighting the importance of finding a balance between the two.The book provides insightful recommendations for policymakers, business leaders, and other stakeholders on how to promote public health while maintaining economic resilience. The authors have approached the topic from various perspectives, providing a multidimensional understanding of the issue and offering practical solutions that can be implemented in real-world scenarios.

I believe this book is a valuable resource for anyone interested in the intersection of public health and economic resilience, and I highly recommend it to policymakers, business leaders, academics, and anyone concerned about the future of our society.

Dr. Bharath J

Preface

Public Health and Economic Resilience: Implications for Business, Government, and Society is a timely and comprehensive book that explores the intersection of public health and economic resilience. The book addresses the need for businesses, governments, and society as a whole to understand the critical role that public health plays in economic stability and growth.The COVID-19 pandemic has highlighted the importance of public health and the urgent need for resilient health systems. This book examines the lessons learned from the pandemic and offers strategies for building more resilient health systems for the future.

The book also discusses the role of businesses in promoting public health and building economic resilience, and explores the ways in which government policies can impact public health and economic growth. It addresses health disparities, the costs and benefits of investing in public health, and the potential for technology and innovation to promote public health.In addition, this book emphasizes the importance of community involvement in promoting public health and building economic resilience. It highlights successful community-driven public health initiatives that can serve as models for future efforts.

This book brings together experts from a wide range of disciplines, including public health, economics, business, and policy. It is intended for anyone interested in understanding the relationship between public health and economic resilience and is an important resource for businesses, government officials, policymakers, and public health professionals.We hope this book provides valuable insights into the critical role of public health in building a more resilient future for us all.

Sincerely,

Dr Bharath J

Acknowledgements

Writing a book requires the support and assistance of many people, and we would like to take this opportunity to express our gratitude to those who have contributed to this project.First and foremost, we would like to thank the contributors of this book for their valuable insights and perspectives on the intersection of public health and economic resilience. Your expertise and dedication have made this book possible, and we are honored to have had the opportunity to work with you.We would also like to extend our appreciation to our colleagues, friends, and family members who have supported us throughout the writing process. Your encouragement, feedback, and patience have been invaluable.

Special thanks go to our editors and publishers for their guidance and expertise in bringing this book to fruition. Your hard work and commitment have been instrumental in ensuring that this book meets the highest standards of quality and excellence.Finally, we would like to express our deepest gratitude to the frontline workers and public health officials who have tirelessly worked to keep our communities safe and healthy during these challenging times. Your dedication and sacrifice have inspired us, and we hope that this book will contribute to the ongoing conversation about the importance of public health and economic resilience.

Thank you all for your contributions to this book and for your ongoing commitment to the health and well-being of our communities.

Prologue

The world was caught off-guard in 2020 when the COVID-19 pandemic brought unprecedented disruptions to public health and the global economy. The pandemic exposed the fragility of health systems, and the interconnectedness of public health and economic resilience. It also highlighted the urgent need for businesses, governments, and society to work together to address the challenges posed by the pandemic.

As we navigate the post-pandemic world, the importance of public health and economic resilience has become even more apparent. The challenges we face require a multi-disciplinary and collaborative approach, with a focus on building resilience and promoting equity.

This book, "Public Health and Economic Resilience: Implications for Business, Government, and Society," brings together experts from diverse fields to explore the intersections of public health and economic resilience. Through a series of chapters, we examine the relationship between public health and economic stability, discuss the challenges and opportunities faced by businesses and governments in promoting public health, and explore strategies for building a more resilient future.

We hope that this book will spark new conversations and collaborations, and inspire innovative approaches to promoting public health and economic resilience. Together, we can build a more resilient and equitable future.

CHAPTER I

Introduction: The Intersection of Public Health and Economic Resilience

The COVID-19 pandemic has brought to light the interconnectedness of public health and economic resilience. The pandemic has not only caused massive disruptions to health systems worldwide but has also severely impacted economies, leading to job losses, business closures, and economic instability. This situation highlights the need for a better understanding of the relationship between public health and economic resilience and the importance of maintaining this balance.

This chapter will provide an overview of the book and introduce the key concepts of public health and economic resilience. It will also discuss why these concepts are important for businesses, governments, and society as a whole.

Overview of the Book

The book aims to explore the intersection of public health and economic resilience and its implications for businesses, governments, and society. It consists of ten chapters that examine various aspects of this relationship and how it affects different sectors.

1. Introduction: The Intersection of Public Health and Economic Resilience, This current chapter will provide an overview of the book and introduce the key concepts of public health and economic resilience. It will also

discuss why these concepts are important for businesses, governments, and society as a whole.

2. Public Health and Economic Resilience: What's the Connection? This chapter will explore the relationship between public health and economic resilience, and highlight how public health can contribute to economic stability and growth. It will also discuss the economic consequences of poor public health.
3. Building Resilient Health Systems: Lessons from the COVID-19 Pandemic, This chapter will examine how the COVID-19 pandemic has highlighted the importance of resilient health systems, and explore strategies for building more resilient health systems in the future.
4. Business Resilience and Public Health: Challenges and Opportunities, This chapter will discuss the role of businesses in promoting public health and building economic resilience, and highlight examples of businesses that have successfully integrated public health into their operations.
5. Government Policy and Public Health: Navigating the Intersections, This chapter will explore the ways in which government policies can impact public health and economic resilience, and discuss the challenges of balancing economic growth with public health goals.
6. Economic Resilience and Health Equity: Addressing Disparities in Public Health, This chapter will discuss the ways in which health disparities can impact economic resilience, and explore strategies for addressing these disparities and promoting health equity.
7. Investing in Public Health: Costs, Benefits, and Trade-Offs This chapter will explore the costs and benefits

of investing in public health, and discuss, the trade-offs that businesses, governments, and society must consider when making decisions about public health investments.

8. Technology, Innovation, and Public Health: Opportunities and Challenges, This chapter will explore the potential for technology and innovation to promote public health and economic resilience, and discuss the challenges and ethical considerations associated with these developments.
9. The Role of Communities in Public Health and Economic Resilience, This chapter will discuss the role of communities in promoting public health and building economic resilience, and highlight examples of successful community-driven public health initiatives.
10. Conclusion Building a Resilient Future, This chapter will summarize the key themes of the book and offer suggestions for how businesses, governments, and society can work together to build a more resilient future that prioritizes public health and economic stability.

Key Concepts

Public health is a field that encompasses a range of activities aimed at promoting and protecting the health of populations. It includes disease surveillance, vaccination campaigns, and healthcare system management. Public health measures are essential for controlling the spread of infectious diseases and preventing non-communicable diseases such as cancer and heart disease. Public health also includes efforts to promote healthy behaviors such as physical activity and healthy eating.

Economic resilience refers to the ability of an economic system to withstand and recover from shocks and stresses. Economic shocks can come from various sources, such as natural disasters, economic downturns, and geopolitical events. Resilience involves preparing for and adapting to these shocks, including measures such as diversifying the economy, building infrastructure, and promoting innovation. Economic resilience is essential for maintaining economic stability and promoting long-term growth.

Importance of Public Health and Economic Resilience
The COVID-19 pandemic has highlighted the importance of public health measures in controlling the spread of the virus and protecting populations. At the same time, the pandemic has had significant economic impacts, with many businesses closing and economies contracting. The pandemic has demonstrated how public health and economic resilience are closely intertwined, and the need for collaboration between businesses, governments, and society to address these issues effectively.

Public health and economic resilience are also important for businesses. Companies that invest in employee wellness programs can reduce healthcare costs and increase productivity. Investing in public health measures can also help companies to reduce the risk of business interruption due to pandemics or other public health emergencies. In addition, companies that prioritize sustainability and environmental responsibility can improve their reputation and attract customers who are concerned about public health and environmental issues.

Governments also play a critical role in promoting public health and economic resilience. Governments can invest in healthcare infrastructure, disease surveillance networks, and public health campaigns. They can also regulate environmental pollution to protect public health and promote economic resilience. Governments can also incentivize businesses to invest in public health measures by offering tax breaks or other financial incentives.

Challenges and Opportunities

Despite the critical importance of public health and economic resilience, there are several challenges that must be addressed. One significant challenge is the lack of coordination between public health and economic policy. Historically, these two fields have been treated as separate domains, with little overlap in terms of policy and decision-making. Another challenge is the lack of investment in public health infrastructure, which can make it difficult to respond effectively to pandemics and other public health emergencies.

CHAPTER II

Public Health and Economic Resilience: What's the Connection?

India, one of the world's fastest-growing economies, has made significant progress in economic development over the past few decades. However, it still faces a range of public health challenges that have significant economic consequences. This chapter will explore the relationship between public health and economic resilience in the Indian context, highlighting the ways in which public health can contribute to economic stability and growth. We will also discuss the economic consequences of poor public health and the need for investments in public health to promote economic resilience.

The Connection between Public Health and Economic Resilience

Public health is critical for economic resilience, as healthy populations are more productive and better able to participate in the labor force. In India, public health issues such as malnutrition, infectious diseases, and non-communicable diseases have a significant impact on the workforce and the economy. Malnutrition and infectious diseases can lead to increased healthcare costs, reduced productivity, and missed days of work, while non-communicable diseases such as diabetes and cardiovascular disease can lead to premature death and disability, reducing the labor force and economic growth.

Investing in Public Health for Economic Resilience Investments in public health can help to promote economic resilience by reducing healthcare costs, improving productivity, and increasing workforce participation. In India, investments in public health can take many forms, including improvements to healthcare infrastructure, expansion of health insurance coverage, and public health education campaigns. Additionally, investments in preventive measures such as vaccinations, disease screening, and health promotion programs can help to reduce the incidence and impact of diseases on the workforce and the economy.

The Economic Consequences of Poor Public Health

Poor public health can have a significant impact on the economy, as it can result in increased healthcare costs, reduced productivity, and missed days of work. In India, the burden of disease is significant, with many preventable and treatable diseases affecting the population. The economic costs of poor public health in India are estimated to be significant, with studies suggesting that the direct and indirect costs of non-communicable diseases alone could reach 6.2% of GDP by 2030.

The impact of air pollution on health and the economy: India is known for having some of the highest levels of air pollution in the world, particularly in its major cities. This not only has significant public health implications, but it also has economic consequences. For example, a study by the World Bank found that air pollution costs India the equivalent of 8.5% of its GDP each year due to lost productivity, healthcare costs, and other factors.

The role of healthcare access in economic growth: In India, access to healthcare is often limited, particularly for those living in rural areas. This can have significant economic consequences, as poor health can lead to decreased productivity and increased healthcare costs. By investing in public health initiatives and improving access to healthcare, India can promote economic growth and stability.

The impact of infectious disease outbreaks on tourism: India's tourism industry is an important contributor to its economy, but infectious disease outbreaks such as the recent COVID-19 pandemic can have a significant impact on tourism. For example, the cancellation of international flights and the imposition of travel restrictions has led to a significant decline in tourism revenue in India. By effectively responding to public health emergencies and minimizing their impact, India can promote economic resilience in its tourism industry.

The connection between sanitation and economic growth: Poor sanitation is a significant public health issue in India, particularly in rural areas. However, it also has economic consequences. For example, the World Bank estimates that India loses approximately 6.4% of its GDP each year due to the effects of inadequate sanitation, including healthcare costs and lost productivity. By investing in sanitation infrastructure and promoting better hygiene practices, India can improve public health outcomes and promote economic growth.

These examples highlight the close relationship between public health and economic resilience in India. By effectively addressing public health challenges, India can promote economic stability and growth, while also improving the health and well-being of its citizens.

Conclusion Public health is critical for economic resilience, and investments in public health can help to promote economic stability and growth. In India, public health challenges such as malnutrition, infectious diseases, and non-communicable diseases have a significant impact on the workforce and the economy. By investing in public health infrastructure, expanding health insurance coverage, and promoting preventive measures, India can build greater economic resilience and ensure a healthy and productive population.

CHAPTER III

Building Resilient Health Systems: Lessons from the COVID-19 Pandemic

The COVID-19 pandemic has had a profound impact on the world, highlighting the vulnerabilities of global health systems and the urgent need to build more resilient health systems. The pandemic has challenged health systems across the globe, with many countries struggling to respond to the rapidly evolving crisis. This chapter will explore the lessons learned from the COVID-19 pandemic and identify strategies for building more resilient health systems in the future.

The Importance of Resilient Health Systems:

Resilient health systems are essential for responding to public health crises such as the COVID-19 pandemic. A resilient health system is one that is able to withstand shocks and stresses, adapt to changing circumstances, and maintain essential health services during a crisis. In the context of the COVID-19 pandemic, resilient health systems are essential for controlling the spread of the virus, providing care for patients, and supporting public health efforts.

Lessons Learned from the COVID-19 Pandemic:

The COVID-19 pandemic has exposed the weaknesses and vulnerabilities of global health systems, highlighting the need for greater investment in public health and healthcare infrastructure. The following are some of the key lessons learned from the pandemic:

Importance of Early Detection and Rapid Response: Early detection and rapid response are critical for controlling the spread of infectious diseases. The COVID-19 pandemic has highlighted the importance of early detection and rapid response, including rapid testing, contact tracing, and isolation of infected individuals.

Need for Robust Healthcare Infrastructure: The pandemic has exposed the weaknesses in healthcare infrastructure, including shortages of medical supplies and equipment, inadequate staffing levels, and limited hospital capacity. Building a robust healthcare infrastructure that can respond to the needs of the population is essential for building resilient health systems.

Importance of Data and Information Sharing: Effective response to public health crises requires access to accurate and timely data. The COVID-19 pandemic has highlighted the importance of data and information sharing, including sharing information about the spread of the virus, treatment outcomes, and the effectiveness of public health interventions.

Importance of Community Engagement: Community engagement is critical for ensuring that public health measures are effective and sustainable. The COVID-19 pandemic has highlighted the importance of engaging communities in public health efforts, including promoting healthy behaviors, providing accurate information, and addressing concerns and fears.

Strategies for Building Resilient Health Systems:

The COVID-19 pandemic has highlighted the urgent need to build more resilient health systems. The following are some strategies for building resilient health systems:

Investment in Public Health: Investing in public health infrastructure, including surveillance systems, laboratory capacity, and healthcare workforce training, is essential for building resilient health systems.

Strengthening Healthcare Infrastructure: Strengthening healthcare infrastructure, including increasing hospital capacity, ensuring an adequate supply of medical equipment and supplies, and improving staffing levels, is critical for building resilient health systems.

Improving Data and Information Systems: Improving data and information systems, including developing better data collection tools, sharing data across organizations and sectors, and improving data analytics, is essential for building resilient health systems.

Community Engagement and Empowerment: Engaging and empowering communities, including providing education and information, promoting healthy behaviors, and involving communities in decision-making processes, is critical for building resilient health systems.

The COVID-19 pandemic has had a profound impact on the world, highlighting the importance of building resilient health systems that can respond to public health crises. Building resilient health systems requires investment in public health infrastructure, strengthening healthcare infrastructure, improving data and information systems, and engaging and empowering communities. By taking these steps, we can build a more resilient and responsive healthcare system that is better able to protect the health of populations around the world.

CHAPTER IV

Business Resilience and Public Health: Challenges and Opportunities

India has a large and diverse economy with millions of small, medium, and large enterprises. These businesses are a critical part of India's economic growth and development. However, they are also vulnerable to a range of risks, including economic instability, natural disasters, and pandemics.

The COVID-19 pandemic has shown that businesses need to be resilient and adaptable to survive and thrive in challenging times. The pandemic has disrupted supply chains, reduced demand for goods and services, and forced businesses to adopt new ways of working. Businesses that were able to adapt quickly and implement measures to protect the health and safety of their employees and customers were better positioned to weather the storm.

The Role of Businesses in Promoting Public Health in India

Businesses have an important role to play in promoting public health in India. By investing in public health initiatives, businesses can help to prevent the spread of disease, protect the health and safety of their employees and customers, and contribute to the overall health and well-being of the communities in which they operate.

There are several ways in which businesses in India can promote public health. For example, they can provide access to clean drinking water and sanitation facilities for their employees and the surrounding community. They can also promote healthy lifestyles by encouraging physical activity and providing healthy food options in their workplaces.

Additionally, businesses can invest in healthcare infrastructure and services in the communities where they operate. For example, they can provide health education programs, and support vaccination campaigns.

Challenges to Integrating Public Health into Business Operations in India

Despite the potential benefits of integrating public health into business operations, there are several challenges that need to be addressed in India. These challenges include:

One of the major challenges is the limited awareness and understanding of the importance of public health among businesses. Many businesses may not be aware of the potential benefits of investing in public health initiatives or may not understand how to effectively integrate public health into their operations.

Another challenge is the lack of funding and resources to invest in public health initiatives. Many businesses, especially small and medium-sized enterprises, may not have the financial resources to invest in public health initiatives, which can limit their ability to promote public health in their communities.

The fragmented healthcare infrastructure and services in many parts of the country also pose a challenge. Limited access to healthcare services for marginalized communities and rural areas can make it difficult for businesses to effectively promote public health in these areas.

Moreover, limited government support and incentives for businesses to invest in public health initiatives can also be a challenge. The government can play a crucial role in providing support and incentives to businesses that invest in public health, which can encourage more businesses to take action.

Overall, promoting public health in India requires a collaborative effort from businesses, governments, and communities. By addressing the challenges and working together, we can create a healthier and more resilient India.

CHAPTER V

Government Policy and Public Health: Navigating the Intersections

India is a rapidly developing country with a complex set of challenges related to public health and economic development. Government policies play a key role in navigating the intersection of these two critical issues, and the COVID-19 pandemic has further highlighted the need for effective policy responses to public health crises. In this chapter, we will explore the ways in which government policies can impact public health and economic resilience in India, and discuss the challenges of balancing economic growth with public health goals.

Government Policies and Public Health:

The Indian government has taken significant steps to improve public health in recent years, including the introduction of the Ayushman Bharat scheme, which aims to provide health insurance coverage to the country's most vulnerable citizens. However, there are still many challenges to be addressed, particularly in the areas of healthcare infrastructure and access to healthcare services. In order to promote public health and build economic resilience, the government must focus on policies that prioritize health equity and address the root causes of health disparities.

One example of a government policy that has had a significant impact on public health in India is the Swachh Bharat Abhiyan, a campaign launched in 2014 to improve sanitation and hygiene throughout the country. The campaign has led to significant improvements in sanitation and has contributed to a reduction in communicable diseases such as diarrhea and cholera. However, the campaign has also faced challenges in implementation, particularly in rural areas where access to sanitation facilities is limited.

Balancing Economic Growth with Public Health Goals:

In India, as in many other countries, there is often tension between economic growth and public health goals. Policies that promote economic growth, such as industrialization and urbanization, can have negative impacts on public health if not managed carefully. For example, the rapid growth of cities in India has led to increased air pollution, which is a major contributor to respiratory diseases such as asthma and chronic obstructive pulmonary disease (COPD).

At the same time, policies that prioritize public health can also have economic benefits. For example, investments in healthcare infrastructure and disease prevention can lead to improved productivity and reduced healthcare costs over the long term. Policies that address the social determinants of health, such as poverty and education, can also contribute to economic growth by improving human capital and reducing social inequalities.

Government policies play a critical role in promoting public health and building economic resilience in India. The COVID-19 pandemic has highlighted the importance of effective policy responses to public health crises, and has demonstrated the need for policies that balance economic growth with public health goals. Moving forward, the Indian government must continue to prioritize policies that address the root causes of health disparities and promote health equity, while also promoting economic growth in a sustainable and equitable manner. By doing so, India can build a more resilient and prosperous future for all its citizens.

CHAPTER VI

Economic Resilience and Health Equity: Addressing Disparities in Public Health

Health disparities and inequalities have been a persistent issue in India. The country faces a high burden of communicable and non-communicable diseases, which disproportionately affects certain populations based on factors such as socio-economic status, gender, caste, and geography. These disparities not only have a negative impact on the health and well-being of individuals but also pose significant challenges to the economic resilience of the country. This chapter will explore the ways in which health disparities can impact economic resilience in India and discuss strategies for addressing these disparities and promoting health equity.

The Burden of Health Disparities in India India is home to one-fifth of the world's population, and yet it accounts for a disproportionately high burden of communicable and non-communicable diseases. According to the World Health Organization (WHO), India accounts for 27% of global tuberculosis cases, 40% of the global burden of dengue, and 60% of the world's leprosy cases. Furthermore, non-communicable diseases such as diabetes, cardiovascular diseases, and cancer are on the rise, and these diseases disproportionately affect the urban poor and rural populations.

Health disparities in India are closely linked to socio-economic status, with those from lower-income backgrounds experiencing greater health inequities. For example, the infant mortality rate in India is 28 per 1,000 live births, but in some of the poorest states, it can be as high as 43 per 1,000 live births. Similarly, the maternal mortality ratio in India is 97 per 100,000 live births, but in some states, it is as high as 195 per 100,000 live births. These disparities are also evident in access to healthcare services, with the poorest segments of the population having limited access to quality healthcare.

The Impact of Health Disparities on Economic Resilience The impact of health disparities on economic resilience in India is significant. Poor health outcomes among disadvantaged populations can lead to decreased productivity, increased healthcare costs, and a reduced ability to participate in the workforce. This not only has implications for individual well-being but also affects the economic development of the country.

In addition, health disparities can contribute to a cycle of poverty, as individuals from disadvantaged backgrounds are more likely to experience poor health outcomes, which can lead to reduced income and limited access to healthcare services. This can further exacerbate health inequities and contribute to economic instability.

Strategies for Addressing Health Disparities and Promoting Health Equity Addressing health disparities in India requires a multi-faceted approach that involves improving access to healthcare services, addressing social determinants of health, and promoting health equity. The following strategies can be implemented to address health disparities and promote health equity:

1. Strengthening primary healthcare: The primary healthcare system in India needs to be strengthened

to improve access to healthcare services, particularly in rural areas. This can be achieved by increasing the number of healthcare providers, improving the quality of healthcare services, and expanding the reach of healthcare services.

2. Addressing social determinants of health: Social determinants of health such as poverty, education, and housing play a significant role in determining health outcomes. Addressing these determinants can help reduce health disparities and promote health equity. Strategies such as increasing access to education, improving housing conditions, and providing social safety nets can help address social determinants of health.
3. Promoting preventive care: Promoting preventive care can help reduce the burden of disease and prevent health disparities. This can be achieved through initiatives such as vaccination programs, health education campaigns, and screening programs.
4. Improving healthcare financing: Healthcare financing in India is fragmented, with limited access to health

CHAPTER VII

Investing in Public Health: Costs, Benefits, and Trade-Offs

Public health investments are often seen as a cost rather than a benefit, especially in developing countries like India. However, public health is a critical component of economic development and resilience. Investing in public health can not only prevent disease outbreaks and save lives, but it can also boost economic growth by improving workforce productivity, reducing healthcare costs, and attracting investment. This chapter will explore the costs and benefits of investing in public health and discuss the trade-offs that businesses, governments, and society must consider when making decisions about public health investments.

Costs of Poor Public Health

The costs of poor public health can be significant, both in terms of human suffering and economic impact. India is one of the countries with the highest burden of disease globally, and the cost of this burden is enormous. Poor public health can result in increased healthcare costs, decreased productivity, and reduced economic growth. It can also lead to increased poverty and inequality, as the poor are often the most vulnerable to the health impacts of environmental degradation and poor living conditions.

Benefits of Investing in Public Health

Investing in public health can bring many benefits to individuals, communities, and societies. Improved public health can reduce healthcare costs by preventing diseases and reducing the need for medical treatment. It can also improve workforce productivity by reducing absenteeism and improving overall health. Additionally, public health interventions can attract investment, as healthy communities are more attractive to businesses looking to establish operations.

In India, the benefits of investing in public health can be seen in the success of the polio eradication campaign. The government invested heavily in the campaign, and as a result, India was declared polio-free in 2014. This achievement not only prevented thousands of cases of disability and death but also demonstrated India's commitment to public health and its ability to successfully implement large-scale public health interventions.

Trade-Offs in Public Health Investments

Despite the many benefits of investing in public health, there are also trade-offs that must be considered. Public health investments require resources that could be used for other priorities, such as education or infrastructure. There may also be trade-offs between short-term and long-term benefits, as some public health interventions may take time to show results.

Another challenge is the trade-off between prevention and treatment. While prevention is often more cost-effective in the long run, it may require more significant upfront investments. In contrast, treatment may provide immediate benefits but can be costly over time.

Strategies for Investing in Public Health

Investing in public health requires a comprehensive approach that considers the trade-offs and benefits of different interventions. One strategy is to prioritize investments in prevention, such as vaccination campaigns, clean water and sanitation, and healthy lifestyle promotion. These interventions can have long-term benefits and be cost-effective in the long run.

Another strategy is to invest in health systems and infrastructure, such as hospitals, clinics, and medical equipment. These investments can improve access to healthcare and provide a foundation for more comprehensive public health interventions.

In India, the government has implemented several public health initiatives, such as the National Health Mission and the Ayushman Bharat program, aimed at improving access to healthcare and reducing the burden of disease. These initiatives demonstrate the government's commitment to public health and can provide a foundation for future investments in public health.

Investing in public health is critical for economic resilience and growth, but it requires careful consideration of costs, benefits, and trade-offs. In India, the government and businesses must work together to prioritize investments in public health and promote health equity. By investing in public health, India can improve the health and well-being of its citizens, reduce healthcare costs, and attract investment, ultimately leading to a more resilient and prosperous society.

1. Costs of neglecting public health: In India, the cost of neglecting public health can be seen in the high burden of preventable diseases like tuberculosis, malaria, and malnutrition. These conditions not only result in high healthcare costs, but also reduce productivity and hinder economic growth. For instance, a study by the World Bank estimated that India lost around $3.3 billion in GDP due to malnutrition in 2017.
2. Benefits of investing in public health: Investing in public health can lead to significant economic benefits, such

as increased productivity and reduced healthcare costs. For example, many studies found that every rupee spent on immunization resulted in a net economic benefit of Rs. 16.5. This is because immunization prevents diseases that can result in lost productivity and healthcare costs.

3. Trade-offs in public health investment: When making decisions about public health investments, there are often trade-offs to consider. For example, investing in preventive measures like vaccination programs can be expensive in the short-term, but can result in significant long-term savings. On the other hand, investing in treatment options for existing health problems may provide more immediate benefits, but may not address the underlying causes of the problem.
4. Role of public-private partnerships: Public-private partnerships (PPPs) can be an effective way to finance public health investments while sharing costs and risks between the public and private sectors. For example, in India, the government has partnered with private companies to finance and implement initiatives like the Swachh Bharat Abhiyan (Clean India Mission) and the Ayushman Bharat health insurance scheme. These partnerships have helped to mobilize resources and expertise from both sectors to address public health challenges.
5. Challenges in public health investment: Despite the potential benefits of investing in public health, there are several challenges that must be addressed. These include limited funding, inadequate infrastructure, and insufficient human resources. In India, for example, the public health system is often underfunded and understaffed, resulting in poor health outcomes and

reduced economic resilience.

By addressing these challenges and investing in public health, India can build a more resilient and prosperous society for all.

CHAPTER VIII

Technology, Innovation, and Public Health: Opportunities and Challenges

Advances in technology and innovation have transformed the way we live, work, and interact with one another. From smartphones to wearables, from telemedicine to artificial intelligence, technology has the potential to revolutionize public health and drive economic growth. In the Indian context, where the healthcare system is underfunded and overburdened, technology and innovation can offer promising solutions to improve health outcomes and promote economic resilience.

However, with these opportunities come challenges and ethical considerations that must be carefully navigated. This chapter will explore the opportunities and challenges associated with technology and innovation in public health, and discuss the Indian context.

Opportunities

Telemedicine is a rapidly growing field in India, and has the potential to address many of the challenges associated with access to healthcare. With a shortage of doctors and healthcare facilities in rural areas, telemedicine can provide remote access to medical expertise, diagnostics, and treatment. It can also reduce the need for patients to travel long distances to receive care, which can be both costly and time-consuming.

The COVID-19 pandemic has highlighted the importance of telemedicine in ensuring continuity of care while reducing the risk of infection. The Indian government has taken steps to promote telemedicine, including issuing guidelines for telemedicine practice and increasing funding for telemedicine infrastructure.

Digital Health Records

Digital health records have the potential to improve healthcare delivery and patient outcomes by providing healthcare providers with real-time access to patient information. This can reduce errors, improve coordination of care, and enable more personalized treatment plans.

In India, where paper-based records are still common, digital health records can help to standardize and streamline healthcare delivery. The government's National Digital Health Mission aims to create a digital health ecosystem that will enable citizens to access their health records, book appointments, and receive teleconsultations.

Artificial Intelligence

Artificial intelligence (AI) has the potential to transform healthcare by enabling faster and more accurate diagnosis, personalized treatment plans, and improved patient outcomes. In India, where the burden of non-communicable diseases such as diabetes and cardiovascular disease is high, AI can help to improve disease management and reduce healthcare costs.

AI-powered technologies such as chatbots and virtual assistants can also help to improve access to healthcare information and support, particularly for those in remote or underserved areas.

Challenges and Ethical Considerations

Data Privacy and Security

The use of technology in healthcare generates large amounts of data, which must be collected, stored, and analyzed. However, this data must be kept secure and confidential to protect patient privacy. In India, where data privacy laws are still evolving, there is a risk of data breaches and misuse of patient information.

The government's Personal Data Protection Bill, which is currently being reviewed, aims to establish a framework for data privacy and security. However, there are concerns about the scope and enforcement of the bill, particularly in relation to the use of data by the government.

Access and Equity

While technology and innovation have the potential to improve access to healthcare, there is a risk of exacerbating existing inequities. For example, those who do not have access to the internet or smartphones may be excluded from digital health initiatives.

There is also a risk of widening the gap between urban and rural areas, where access to technology and healthcare facilities is uneven. The government must ensure that technology and innovation are used in a way that promotes equitable access to healthcare.

Bias and Discrimination

Artificial intelligence and machine learning algorithms are only as unbiased as the data they are trained on. There is a risk that biases and discrimination, whether intentional or unintentional, can be perpetuated through technology and innovation.

Telemedicine has been gaining traction in India, particularly in rural areas where access to healthcare is limited. Telemedicine allows doctors to remotely diagnose and treat patients using video conferencing, mobile apps, and other digital tools. In 2020, the Indian government launched the eSanjeevani telemedicine platform, which has been used by over 1.5 million patients across the country.

However, there are also challenges and ethical considerations associated with the use of technology in public health. One major concern is data privacy and security. The large amounts of health data generated by digital tools must be protected from misuse, and patients must have control over their own data. In addition, there is a risk of exacerbating existing health disparities if certain groups are unable to access or use digital health tools.

Another challenge is ensuring that technology and innovation are used in a way that is equitable and inclusive. For example, some populations may not have access to the necessary digital infrastructure or may not be able to afford digital devices. It is important to consider these factors when developing and implementing technology-based public health interventions.

In conclusion, technology and innovation have the potential to significantly improve public health and economic resilience in India. However, it is important to carefully consider the challenges and ethical considerations associated with these developments and ensure that they are implemented in an equitable and inclusive manner.

CHAPTER IX

The Role of Communities in Public Health and Economic Resilience in India

In India, communities have been integral in promoting public health and building economic resilience. With a population of over 1.3 billion people and significant socio-economic and health disparities, community-driven public health initiatives have played a critical role in addressing health challenges and building economic resilience. This chapter will explore the role of communities in promoting public health and economic resilience in India and highlight examples of successful community-driven public health initiatives.

Community-driven Public Health Initiatives in India Community-driven public health initiatives in India have a long history, with various community organizations playing a critical role in addressing health challenges. In rural areas, non-governmental organizations (NGOs) have played a significant role in providing healthcare services.

Role of Communities in Economic Resilience Communities also play a critical role in building economic resilience. In India, community-based organizations have been instrumental in promoting economic resilience by providing training and employment opportunities to vulnerable groups. For example, the National Rural Livelihoods Mission (NRLM) is a government-led initiative that aims to alleviate poverty by promoting self-employment and entrepreneurship in rural areas. NRLM provides training and financial support to individuals and groups, including women and marginalized communities, to start their businesses. Through their initiatives, NRLM has empowered thousands of individuals and promoted economic resilience in rural areas.

Community participation can be instrumental in improving health outcomes and reducing the economic impact of public health emergencies. For instance, during the COVID-19 pandemic, several communities in India came together to provide essential services such as food and medical supplies to vulnerable populations.

Here are some examples of community-driven public health initiatives in India:

Community health workers: Community health workers, also known as Accredited Social Health Activists (ASHAs), play a crucial role in providing healthcare services to rural and marginalized communities. They work closely with local healthcare facilities and provide information on health issues and preventive measures to community members.

Self-help groups: Self-help groups are community-based organizations that focus on improving the economic and social well-being of their members. These groups can play an important role in promoting public health by educating members on health issues, providing access to healthcare services, and mobilizing resources to address health challenges.

Water and sanitation initiatives: Lack of access to clean water and sanitation facilities is a major public health issue in India. Community-based initiatives such as the Swachh Bharat Mission and the Jal Jeevan Mission aim to provide clean water and sanitation facilities to all households in the country.

Disaster management: India is prone to natural disasters such as floods and earthquakes, which can have a significant impact on public health and economic stability. Community-based disaster management initiatives can help to reduce the impact of disasters by providing emergency response and support services to affected communities.

However, there are also challenges in promoting community-driven public health initiatives in India, such as:

Limited resources: Many communities in India have limited resources and may struggle to invest in public health initiatives.

Limited awareness: Many community members may not be aware of the importance of public health or the services available to them.

Stigma and discrimination: Stigma and discrimination against certain health conditions, such as mental health, can make it difficult to promote public health initiatives within some communities.

Limited government support: There is a need for greater government support and investment in community-driven public health initiatives.

In conclusion, communities in India have a crucial role to play in promoting public health and building economic resilience. By investing in community-driven initiatives, we can ensure that everyone has access to healthcare services and resources, and promote a more equitable and resilient society.

CHAPTER X

Conclusion - Building a Resilient Future

This book has explored the intersection of public health and economic resilience, and the importance of prioritizing both for building a more resilient future. Through examining various aspects of public health, including health systems, business resilience, government policies, health equity, public health investments, technology, innovation, and community engagement, we have seen how these factors are essential for creating a resilient society.

In India, the COVID-19 pandemic has underscored the need for building resilient health systems and economic structures that can withstand shocks and adapt to changing circumstances. The pandemic has brought to light the critical importance of public health infrastructure and the need for strategic investments in healthcare, research, and innovation.

One of the key takeaways from this book is the need for collaboration and cooperation between businesses, governments, and communities to build a resilient future. The private sector has an important role to play in promoting public health and economic resilience, by investing in research and development, implementing effective health and safety measures, and supporting community-based initiatives.

At the same time, governments need to create an enabling environment for businesses to thrive while prioritizing public health goals. This includes developing policies that promote health equity, investing in public health infrastructure, and fostering partnerships with the private sector and civil society.

Community engagement is also essential for building a resilient future. Communities can contribute to promoting public health and economic resilience by supporting local initiatives, advocating for health equity, and participating in decision-making processes.

To build a more resilient future in India, it is crucial to address existing health disparities and promote health equity. This requires a holistic approach that recognizes the social determinants of health, such as poverty, education, and access to healthcare, and implements strategies to address these factors.

Investing in public health is essential for building economic resilience, as healthy populations are more productive and better equipped to adapt to changing circumstances. While there may be costs associated with investing in public health, the benefits far outweigh the costs in the long run.

Finally, technology and innovation have the potential to revolutionize public health and promote economic resilience. However, it is important to ensure that these developments are ethically sound, promote health equity, and prioritize the well-being of communities.

In conclusion, building a resilient future requires a multifaceted approach that prioritizes public health, economic stability, and community engagement. By working together, businesses, governments, and communities can build a future that is better equipped to withstand shocks and adapt to changing circumstances. The time to act is now, and we must seize this opportunity to build a more resilient future for all.

9 798889 864493

Printed by Libri Plureos GmbH in Hamburg,
Germany